Yoga Guide For Starters

Essentials Basics And Techniques

By

Kathy D. Corea

Table Of Contents

Introduction

Yoga is no longer just for yogis. Everywhere you go in many areas of the world, you'll see folks carrying a rolled-up yoga mat over their shoulder. Perhaps you've contemplated joining a class but were put off by these fit, lively people in fitting pants with meditative expressions.

If you want to start moving more but don't know where to start, yoga is a terrific place to start. You can do it anywhere and adjust it to your level as you gain strength and flexibility. It's time to roll out your yoga mat and learn the combination of physical and mental activities that has captivated yoga practitioners all around the world for thousands of years.

The great thing about yoga is that you don't have to be a yogi or yogini to benefit from it. Yoga can soothe the mind and strengthen the body, whether you are young or elderly, overweight or fit. Don't be put off by yoga vocabulary, fancy yoga studios, or difficult positions. Everyone can benefit from yoga.

What Is Yoga, And How Does It Work?

The ancient and intricate practice of yoga has its origins in the Indian school of thought. It was first meant to be a spiritual practice, but more and more people are using it as a way to improve their physical and mental health. Traditional yoga also has other parts, but the styles that are popular in the United States tend to focus on meditative practices, physical poses called asanas, and breathing exercises called pranayama (dyana).
There are many different forms of yoga, ranging from activities that are easy on the body to ones that are more strenuous. Variations in the styles of yoga utilized in research studies might have an impact on the findings of those investigations.

Because of this, conducting an analysis of the studies on the health benefits of yoga is difficult.

Activities such as yoga, tai chi, and qi gong, all of which have their roots in China, are frequently referred to as "meditative movement" practices. In each of these three disciplines, there is a focus on both mental and physical components.

3 Health Benefits Of Yoga

You may be curious about the source of all the excitement. The practice of yoga, on the other hand, has been linked to a wide range of positively significant health effects. The best aspect is that it is not difficult to get started; all you need are a few straightforward workouts. Take a look at some of the following yoga benefits:

A Stronger Mental Attitude And Increased Self-confidence

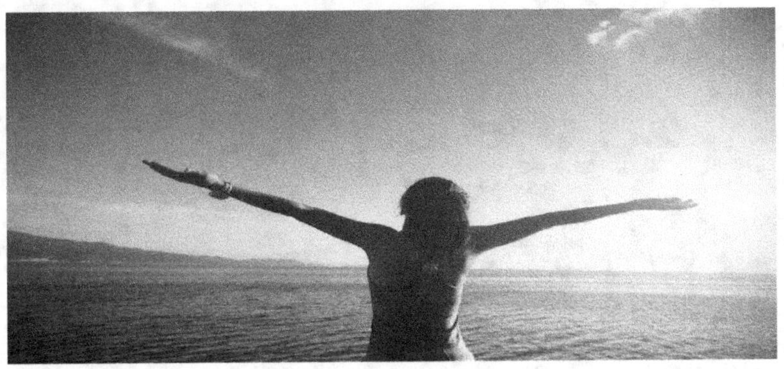

During a yoga session, you should focus solely on yourself and complete the sequence of exercises at your own pace. This is the greatest way to get the most out of your practice. If you are going through a particularly stressful time in your life, practicing yoga can help you calm your racing thoughts and clear your mind so that you can focus on other things.

Increased Strength And Flexibility

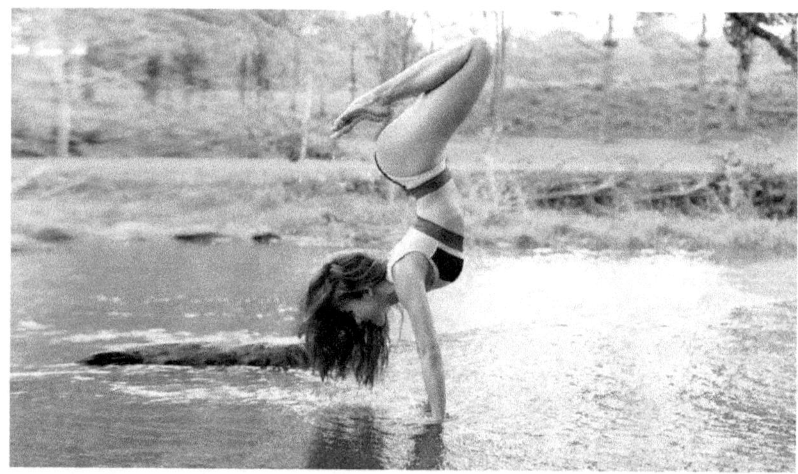

The practice of yoga not only helps bring your body and mind into harmony, but it also helps you become more flexible while increasing your strength. If you spend most of your day sitting, strengthening the muscles in your back is important. Building your core muscles through yoga will not only help you to enhance your posture but will also provide you with more stability for other activities.

Better Sleep And Greater Resilience

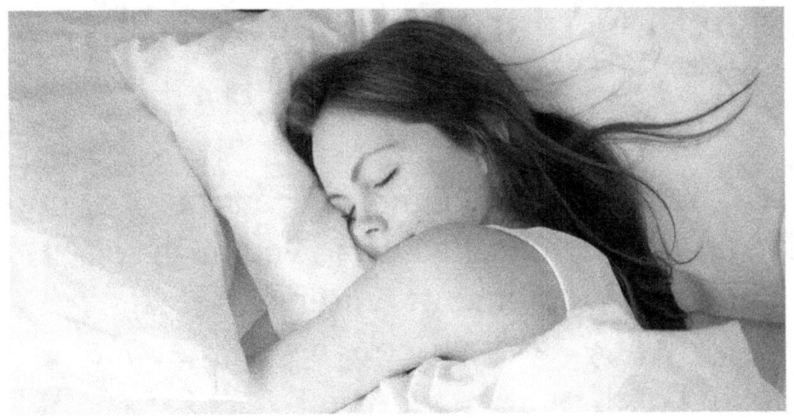

One more significant advantage of doing yoga is that it can help you get a better night's rest. A significant portion of the sessions is devoted to relaxation, and this essentially prepares the body for a restful night's sleep. The more deeply you sleep, the more able you are to withstand the pressures and challenges of day-to-day living.

10 Important Items to Have Before Beginning Your Yoga Practice (Buying Guide)

You'll need some fundamental gear before you can enter the yoga class, and you might also want some supplementary items to supplement your practice. This is what you should purchase.

If you are just starting with your yoga practice, you may not be sure what to anticipate, but rest assured that you have a lot to look forward to in the future. You will be participating in a custom that has been practiced for the past 5,000 years and that has many positive effects on both one's physical and mental well-being.

As you become more proficient in yoga positions, you may look forward to increased strength and flexibility, enhanced quality of sleep, reduced levels of stress, and a healthier heart. You will become a better athlete as a result of all of that.

You will need some fundamental yoga equipment to get started with your yoga practice before entering the yoga studio. To further help you while you learn how to move through a yoga flow, you might wish to invest in some gear designed specifically for yoga as well as one or two yoga accessories that are optional. The following is a list of the yoga equipment that you may find useful to get the most out of your practice.

1. Yoga Mat

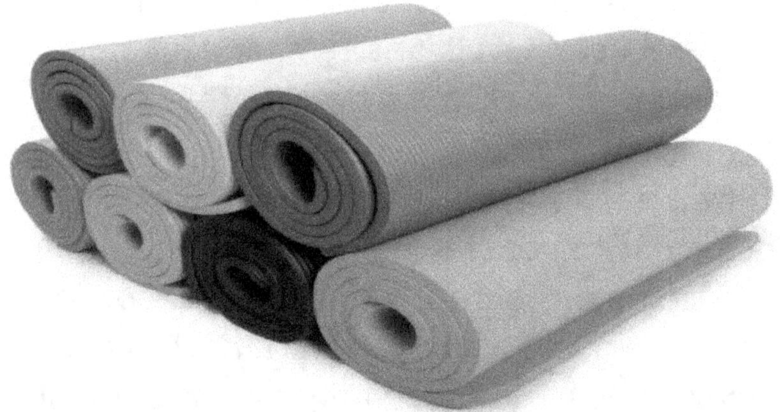

You'll want to have your yoga mat so you can practice discipline at home, and many yoga teachers demand their students bring their mats to class. When you practice a downward-facing dog on a high-quality yoga mat, you will experience improved traction, which will prevent you from falling out of the posture.

A yoga mat will not only act as a layer of padding between your body and the floor, but it will also provide additional support. When looking for a yoga mat that is suitable for your needs, it is important to pay attention to the following considerations regardless of whether you are a novice or an experienced practitioner:

- **Thickness:** A thinner yoga mat offers more support for balance postures, while a thicker yoga mat cushions your bones and joints while you are in poses that bring them into contact with the ground. Standard yoga mats have a thickness of about 3.3 millimeters and offer a nice medium; however, if your practice is more therapeutic in nature, you may want to consider purchasing a mat that is half an inch or an inch and a quarter thick.

Bear in mind that the mat's thickness will also have an effect on how cumbersome it will be for you to transport it.

- **Material:** The materials that were used to manufacture your yoga mat will decide how much traction it offers, how it feels, how long it will last, whether or not it will hold odors, and whether or not it will dry quickly. The vast majority of mats are crafted from PVC or rubber. A natural rubber mat will not only offer traction, but it will also block odors and feel refreshing to the touch. PVC is less friendly to the environment than thermoplastic elastomers and rubber, which is an extra benefit of using these materials. It is recommended that you look for mats that are created from recyclable materials.

2. A Yoga Towel

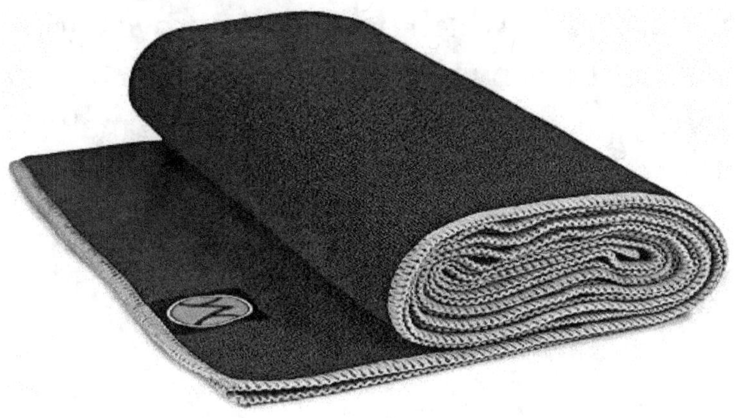

Cover your yoga mat with a yoga towel whenever you participate in a sweat-inducing yoga practice, such as hot yoga, power yoga, or any other style of yoga. This yoga accessory will aid in absorbing sweat, lowering the likelihood of slipping and sustaining an injury during your yoga practice. Rather than using a conventional bath or beach towel, you should invest in a mat towel designed exclusively for yoga.

The vast majority of yoga towels are made from microfibre, which not only improves grip but also reduces bunching. Before class, lightly spritzing your yoga mat with water can make it simpler for your yoga towel to remain in place.

3. Yoga Bag or Sling

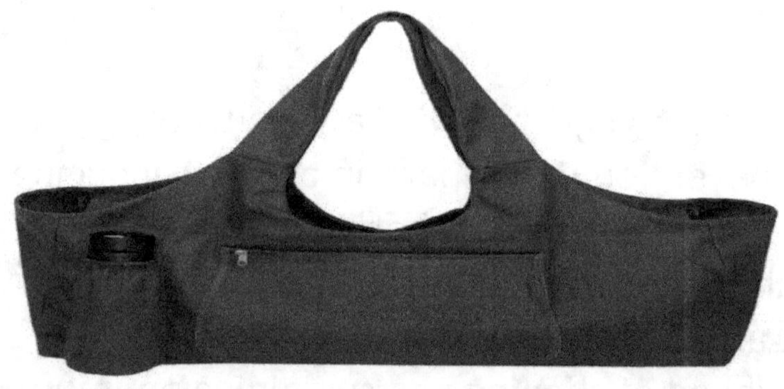

Carrying your yoga mat to and from the studio will likely necessitate either a mat bag or a sling.

A sling is often less expensive, however, a bag has additional compartments for your phone and other requirements.

4. Yoga Blocks

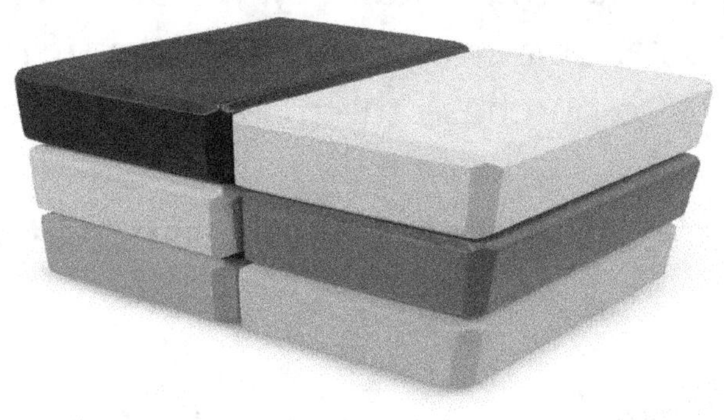

Blocks are an excellent addition for those who lack advanced flexibility since they facilitate the transition into other poses. As your flexibility develops, you may also employ them to deepen a position.

For instance, placing yoga blocks under your hands during a forward fold will provide support if you cannot reach the floor, whereas placing yoga blocks under your feet would challenge you to extend farther to reach the floor.
Select a block with a width of at least four inches for maximum stability. Because some positions require two or three blocks, it is advisable to purchase them as a set.

5. Garments Absolute Necessities for Yoga

When looking for yoga attire, it is of the utmost importance to select garments that are not only comfortable but also able to move with you. This is everything you will need to get started:

- **Pants or Shorts:**

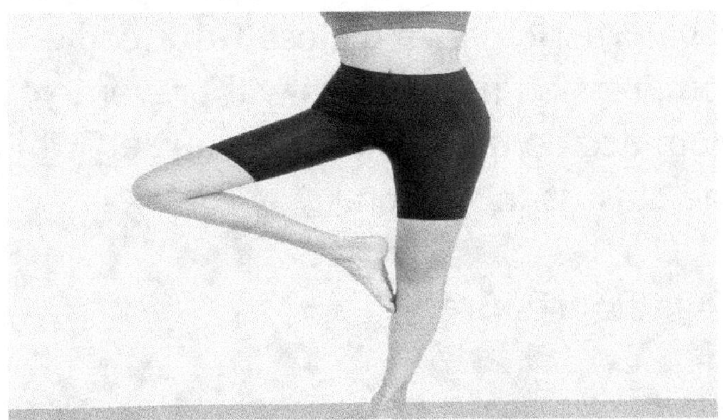

Chose one that can stretch with you and remain in place while you are working out. Whether you choose this route, make sure they are comfortable. You may get the job done with a pair of leggings that have four-way stretch, or you can use a pair of joggers if you want bottoms with a more relaxed fit. Choose a pair of yoga pants with moisture-wicking characteristics, such as those produced with Nike Dri-FIT fabric, if you have a history of perspiring heavily while doing yoga.

Make sure the shorts you choose for your yoga practice have a close fit or come with compression liners. This will prevent you from accidentally exposing yourself while the class is in session.

- **Yoga Sports Bra:**

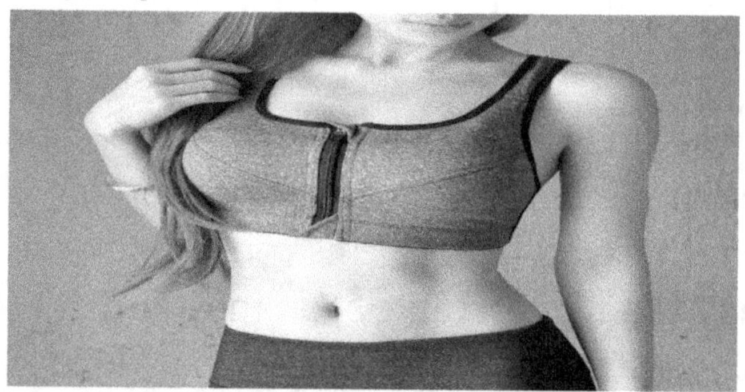

though yoga has a lower impact than many other sports, the majority of women nevertheless choose to wear a light-support or medium-support sports bra when practicing the practice.

- **Tops:**

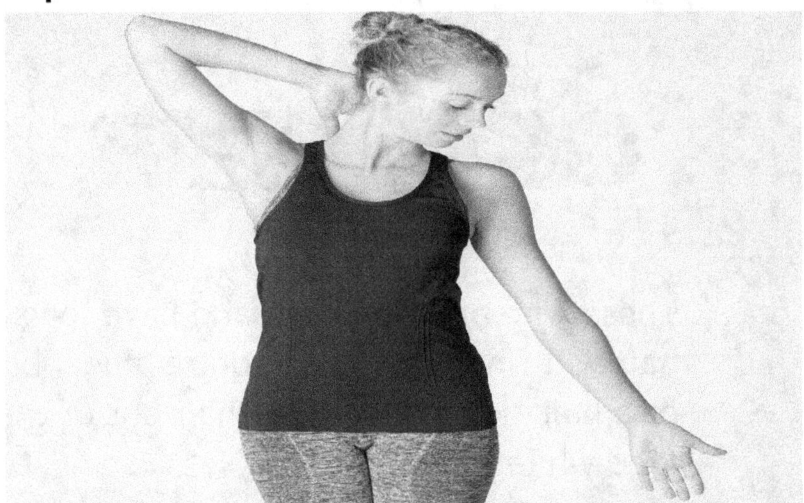

Choose tops that have a form-fitting cut so that you don't end up with your shirt hanging out of your back during an inversion.

• Headband:

Those who practice yoga and have long hair will find that they require a headband or a hair tie to keep their hair out of their face while they move.

• Yoga Socks and Gloves:

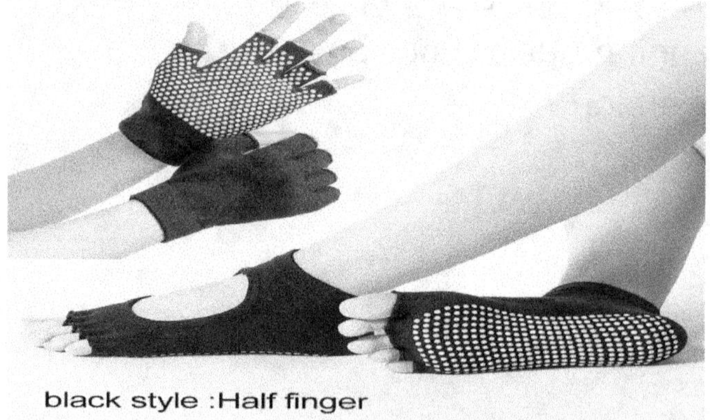

black style :Half finger

Even though most yogis practice without socks or shoes, you might find that wearing a pair of socks designed to provide grip makes you feel more at ease throughout your practice. If you don't have your yoga mat with you while you travel, you'll need a pair of yoga socks and yoga gloves in order to practice on the floor instead of your mat. They will help provide the traction that a yoga mat would, but they won't take up any room in your luggage.

6. Yoga Blankets

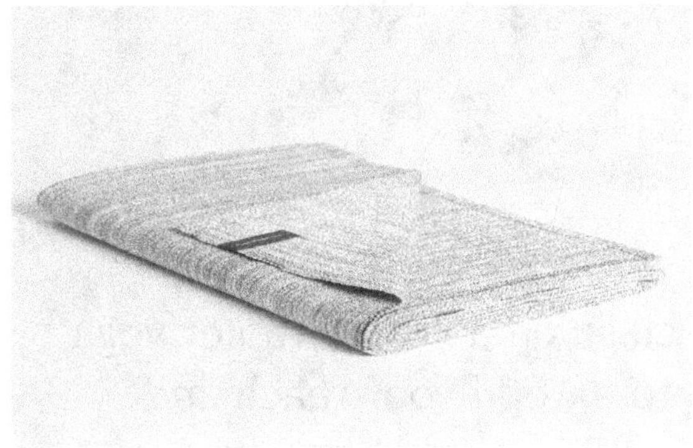

Yoga blankets can offer additional support and cushion for seated or supine poses. You can either purchase a yoga blanket or fold a standard throw blanket at home. You can also use a yoga blanket to cushion your joints, elevate your hips during seated poses, and provide comfort and warmth in the corpse pose or Shavasana.

7. Yoga Straps

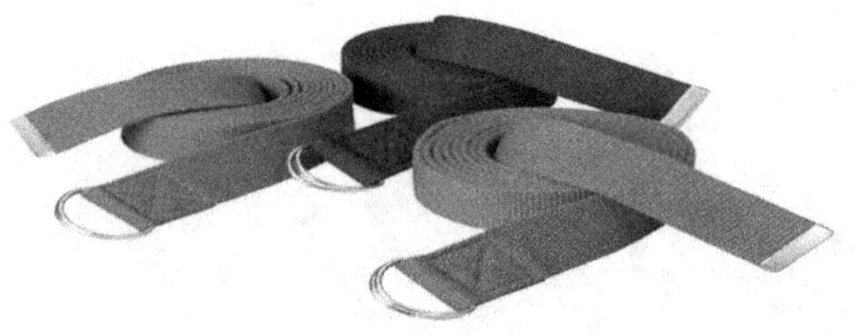

The adjustable clasp on a yoga strap or yoga belt allows you to extend your reach and improve your flexibility and alignment.

For instance, if you cannot reach your feet, a strap is a terrific complement for deepening your seated forward fold. Wrapping the strap over your feet will allow you to pull yourself further into the stretch. If you are unable to clasp your wrists behind your back, straps are also useful for releasing the shoulders. Additionally, they can be utilized for stability and balance in specific poses, such as the boat pose.

8. Impedance Bands

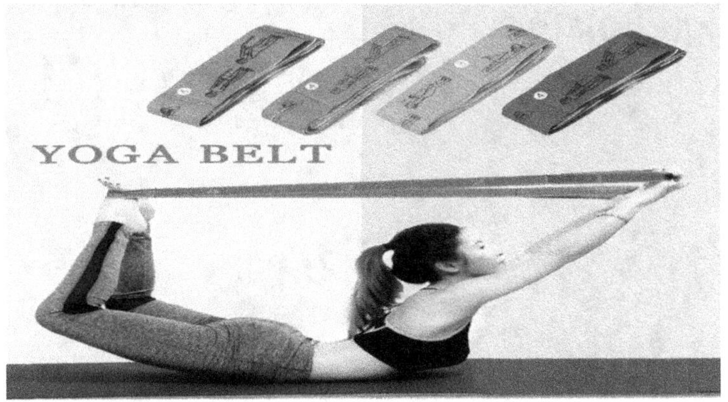

A set of resistance bands can offer an additional level of difficulty to your yoga routine if you wish to maximize your improvements in strength and endurance. According to studies, resistance bands can produce the same strength increases as traditional weights, and they are simpler to include in yoga practice than dumbbells. To target your glutes, you can practice banded donkey kicks while in the table-top pose, for example.

9. Yoga Bolsters

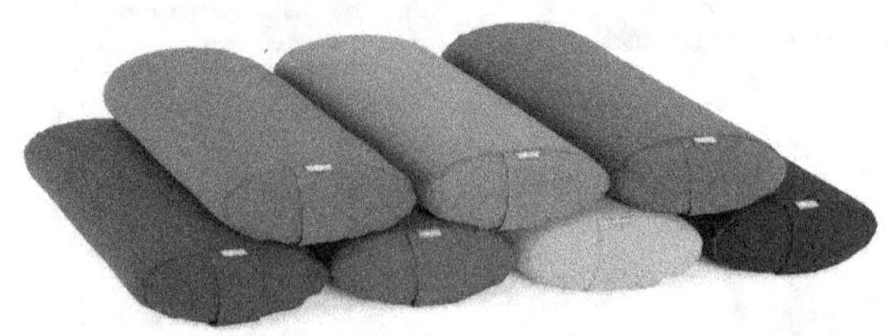

Bolsters give more advanced support than yoga blankets and are useful for therapeutic and pregnant yoga programs in particular. Consider purchasing in both a round and a flat bolster in order to see which best suits your needs. The child's pose can be supported with a bolster, as well as backbends and reclining twists. If you do not frequently require a bolster, a standard pillow or cushion will suffice.

10. Yoga Wheel

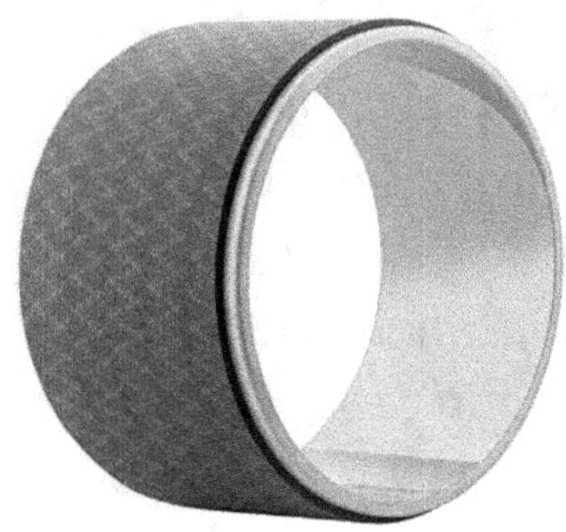

You can use a yoga wheel to support yourself while you are beginning and to push yourself as you advance in your practice. Typical wheel dimensions are 4 inches broad by 12 inches in diameter. In fish pose, a beginner may use a wheel to support their back, neck, and head. As you progress, you can utilize a wheel to make balancing in the crow position or maintaining a plank pose more difficult. Even creative exercises such as rolling lunges and bridges can be performed with a yoga wheel.

Developing an Ambiance

As you develop a home yoga practice, you'll want to cultivate an environment that promotes relaxation and fosters a mind-body connection. You may experiment with the room's temperature, bring in real plants or yoga-inspired artwork that inspires you, or use an essential oil diffuser to produce a pleasant and calming aroma.

As you practice more frequently, you may wish to designate a tranquil spot in your house for meditation.

HOW TO BEGIN THE YOGA PRACTICE

You are probably energized and wondering how you may begin practicing yoga so that you can reap the many benefits it offers. You may perform yoga at home, in a hotel room, on your lunch break at work, or — when you're ready — at a yoga class. This is one of the reasons why so many people choose yoga as a way to get moving since you can do it anywhere and at any time.

If you are having trouble visualizing yourself in a room full of people doing yoga and exposing your lack of flexibility to the world, you should give it a shot in the seclusion and convenience of your own house before going public with it. Take your time, and don't let yourself get sidetracked by the abilities (or lack thereof) of others.

If you are simply concerned with yourself, you will be able to get a better sense of how your body reacts when you perform the various exercises. You won't need much—just some loose-fitting clothes and a yoga mat with non-slip grips will suffice.

16 YOGA POSES FOR BEGINNERS

Always bear in mind the importance of having patience with oneself and maintaining an open mind. In order to get you started with yoga, we have compiled some basic poses for beginners below.

1. Side Plank

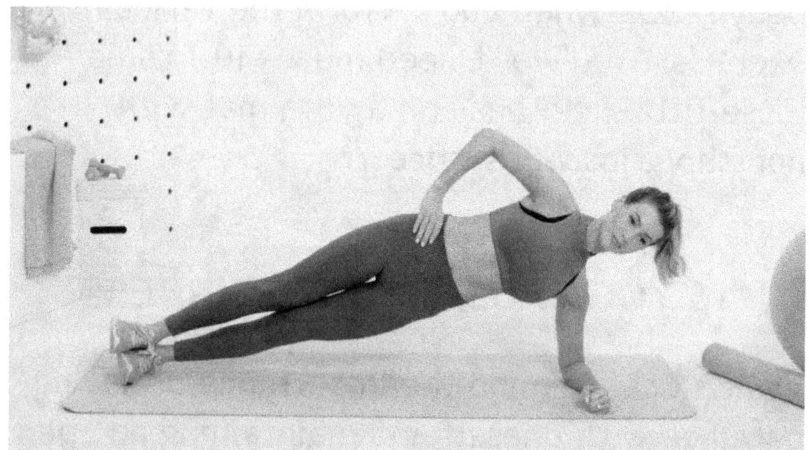

The Side Planks are far more difficult than they appear to be, but the more you do them, the simpler they will become. Placing your forearm on the floor just under your shoulder, stacking your feet on top of each other (or placing one foot in front of the other for added support), and raising your hips until your body is in a straight line are the steps to do the plank position.

If you are just getting started with the plank, you should aim to maintain the posture for 20 or 30 seconds before moving on to the next level.

2. Curl Of The Tiger With a 3-Legged Dog

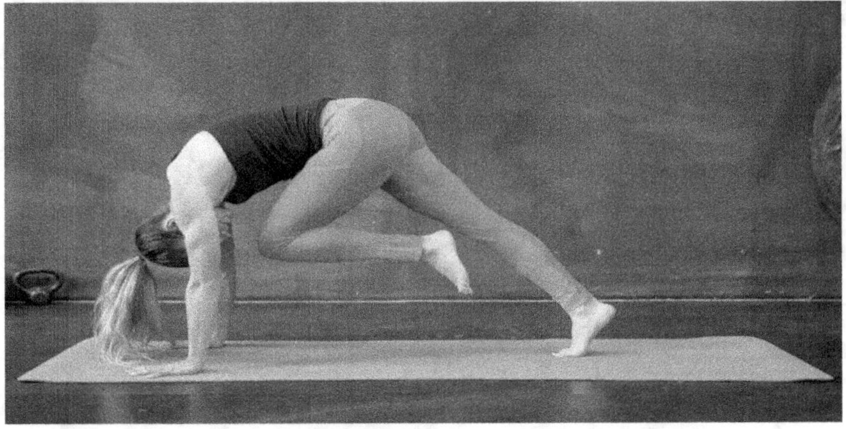

This dynamic action places a significant emphasis on the core as well as the mobility of the entire body, and it is an excellent technique to open up your hips. Begin by getting down on all fours and spreading your hands around the width of your shoulders.

Exhaling, press your palms into the mat and lift your knees till your legs are as straight as possible. Press your palms into the mat. Observe how the back of your legs is stretching out. The "Downward Dog" is one of the most well-known poses for newcomers to try out when they first start practicing yoga. Then, stand on one leg, lift the other leg up straight, and exhale as you bring your knee to your nose. Repeat this with the other leg. Put as much of your belly button as you can into the small of your back, and put as much effort as you can into bringing your knee forward.

3. Warrior III (Three)

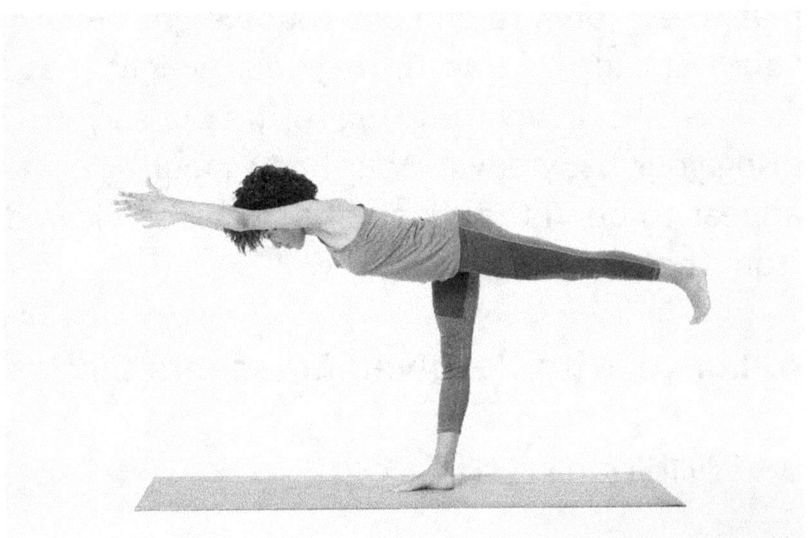

In the Warrior III stance, work on maintaining your balance and concentration while also elongating your spine. To begin, get into a high lunge position by bending your right knee over your right ankle and bringing your palms together in front of your chest. Continue by bending your left leg over your left ankle.

Your left leg is extended behind you in a straight line, and your foot is positioned on the mat. Lean forward and put your weight on your right leg by transferring your weight forward. Raise your left leg to the sky as you bring your body down. Your body should appear to be in the shape of a "T" when viewed from the side.

4. Lunge With Revolved Crescents Circles

Revolved Crescent

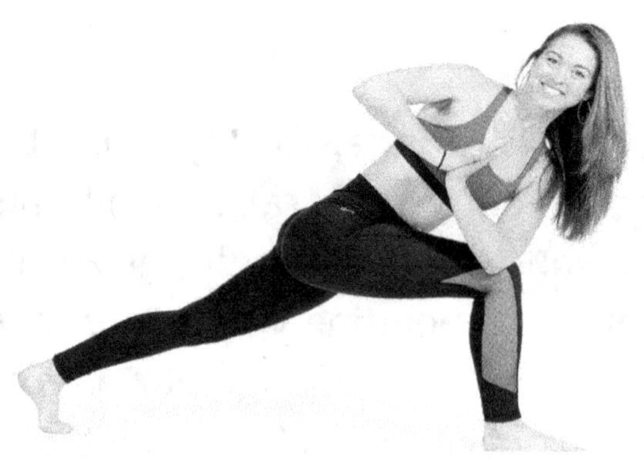

As is the case with other twisting postures, the Revolved Crescent Lunge is beneficial for increasing spine mobility and fostering healthy digestion. Reach your left leg up to the sky as you begin in the Downward Dog position, which is similar to the beginning of the 3-Legged Dog to Tiger Curl seen above. After that, you should step in between your hands and bring your left knee back in toward your nose.

Take a deep breath in and bring your palms together in front of your chest as you elevate your torso into an upright position. Ensure that you are engaging your core muscles and that you are not simply putting all of your weight on your quads. Maintain an active stance on that back leg and focus on driving the back of your right knee up toward the ceiling. Put some forward lean on your torso and connect the outside of your right elbow to the outside of your left leg.

Maintain a long spine while you turn your chest to the left, bringing it closer to the ceiling.

5. Balasana, also known as Child's Pose

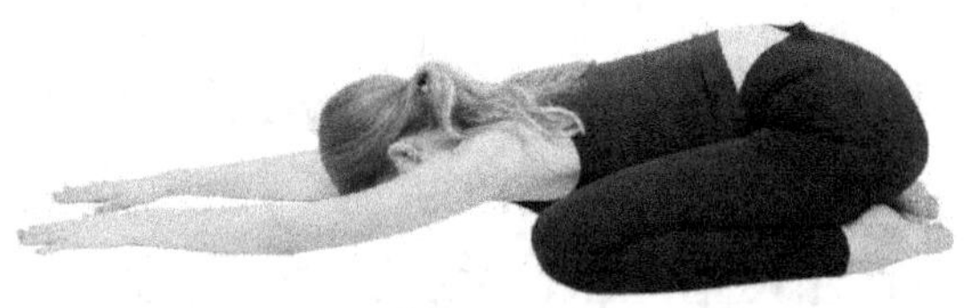

Make a "V" form with your knees by spreading them apart, then bring the tips of your big toes together behind you. Put your buttocks on top of your heels for support. To improve your flexibility, lengthen your spine and stretch forward between your thighs.

You have the option of putting your arms out in front of you or tucking them behind you. This resting pose is an excellent tool for slowing the breath and bringing mental stillness to the practitioner. In addition to this, it stretches your hips and thighs before the beginning of class.

6. Downward-Facing Dog Or Adho Mukha Svanasana

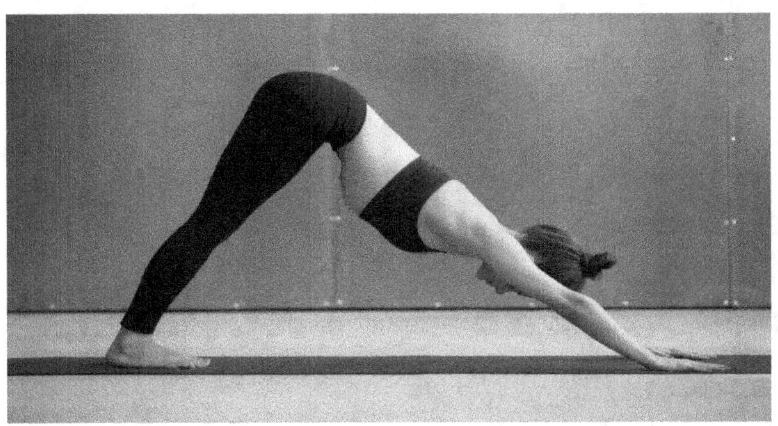

Put your hands and knees on the ground to start (or in cow pose).
Position your hands so that they are under your shoulders, and your knees so that they are under your hips. Your fingertips ought to be pointing toward the very top of the mat.

Spread your fingers apart and make sure that each of your hands is bearing an equal amount of your weight. Raise your knees off the floor and reach your pelvis upward, simulating the action of pulling your hips and thighs backward. It should look like the letter "A" when you stand up straight. Maintain a straight posture, but try not to lock your knees. Relax your neck and look between your knees while you do it.

This position stretches the hamstrings, calves, and spine, which provides the body with a boost of energy.

And you guessed it: the natural stretching motion of a dog is where the term "dog stretch" comes from.

7. Upward-Facing Dog Or Urdhva Mukha Svanasana

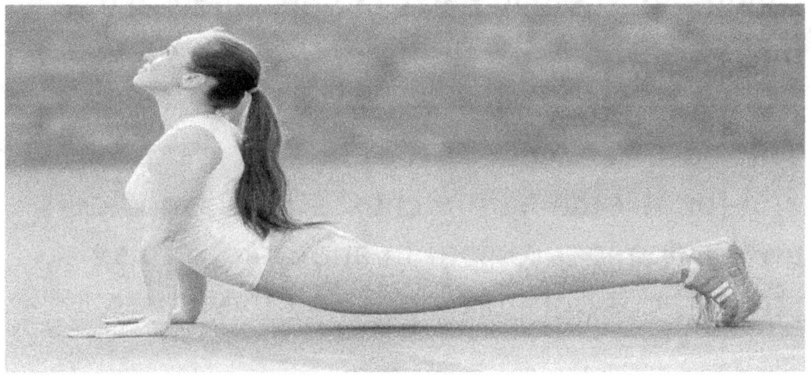

Get started by lying down on your back on your mat. Put some bend in your elbows. Put your hands down on the mat in a sturdy position. Put your fingers further apart.

Your wrists must be positioned such that they are parallel to the mat, and your arms must be held tightly by your sides.

Now, apply pressure all the way through the tops of your feet as you lift your body off the ground. Your hands and the tops of your feet should be the only parts of your body that make contact with the floor. Make a slight arch with your back.
This pose is excellent for enhancing posture and for stretching the chest, lungs, shoulders, and abdominal region. In addition to this, it strengthens both the arms and the wrists.

8. Cobra Or Bhujangasana

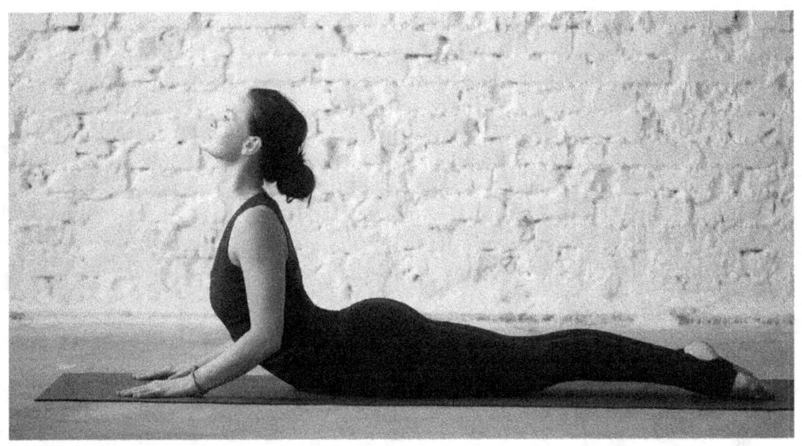

Get started by lying down on your back on your mat. Raise your chest off the ground while you bring your arms into a straight position. Reduce the width of your hips and your legs. Firm your shoulder blades. Put some pressure on the floor with the thighs and the tops of the feet.

The legs and lower torso should remain on the ground in this variation of the dog stance, which is otherwise quite similar to the upward-facing dog.
This yoga stance strengthens the spine while also stretching the lungs, shoulders, and abdominal muscles.

9. Bridge Or Setu Bandha Sarvangasana

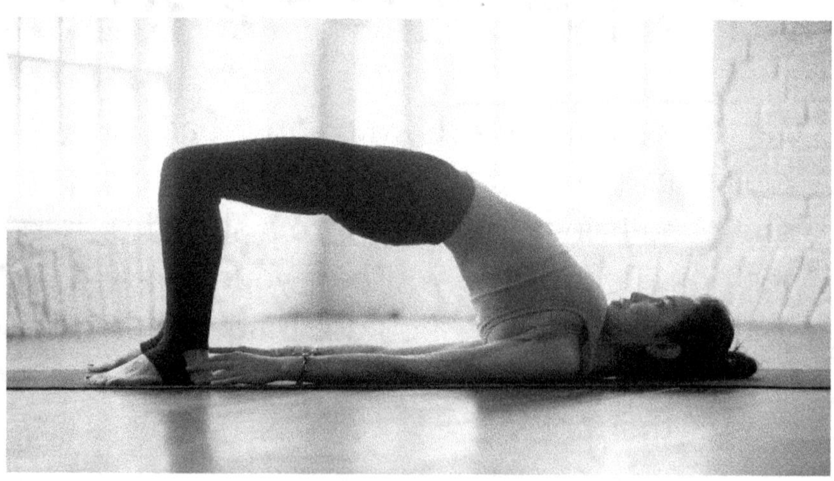

Begin by lying on the floor with your back to the wall and facing the ceiling. Maintain a firm grip on the floor with both your feet and arms as you lift your bottom and upper body off the ground. Your thighs and your feet should be aligned in a parallel fashion. Maintain a position in which the knees are over the heels. You might find it helpful to bring your hands together and clasp them beneath your torso.

This pose is useful for reducing symptoms of exhaustion, headaches, and anxiety. Additionally, it extends the back, as well as the neck and the spine.

10. Chair Pose Or "Utkatasana"

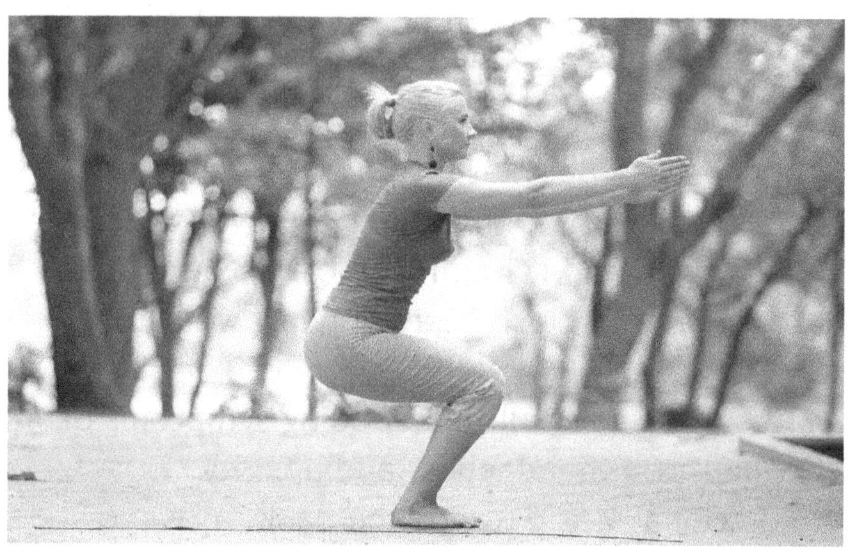

In the Chair position, there is a significant emphasis placed on engaging the legs, back, and abdominal region. Raise both arms directly above your head while bending your knees to the point where your thighs are virtually parallel to the ground.

If you find that you are unable to maintain your arms up, you can either come into cactus arms by bending your arms at the elbows or squeezing your hands together in front of your chest. Bring your hips closer to the floor while keeping your weight on the heels of your feet. You can modify this yoga pose for beginners by placing your back against a wall if you have knee pain while you practice.
The thighs, the calves, and the spine all get a workout from this pose.

11. Warrior One Or Virabhadrasana I

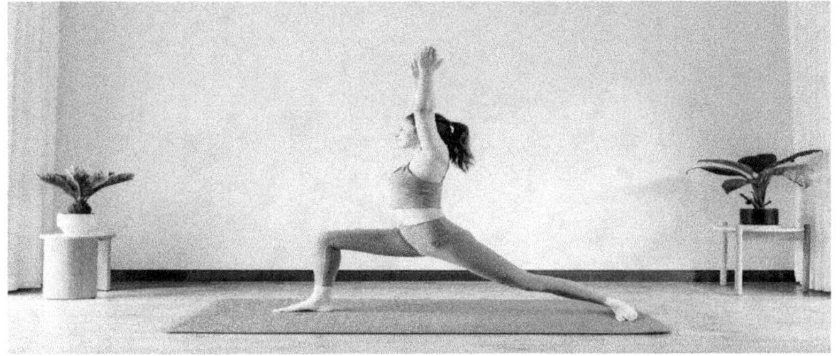

Lean forward on one leg while situating your other leg so that it is parallel to the floor. Your toes should face forward at all times. Your torso should be oriented so that it is facing forward in the direction that you are lunging. Raise your arms to the heavens and let the tension leave your shoulders as you do so. Raise your ribcage toward the ceiling and look forward.

This position stretches the chest as well as the shoulders and the neck, and it also tones the shoulders, arms, thighs, and calves.

12. Warrior Two Or Virabhadrasana II

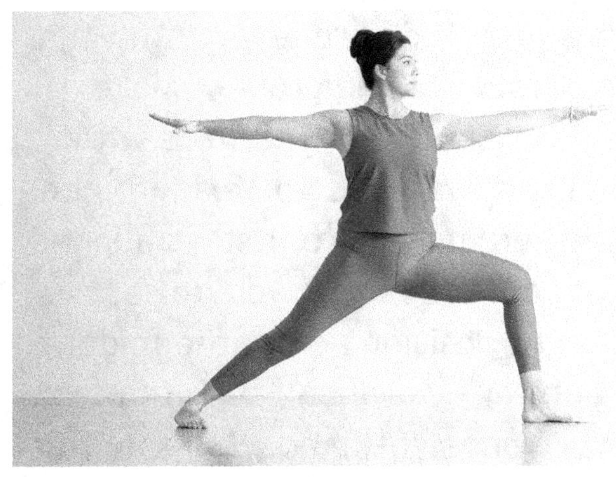

This is a fantastic exercise for developing the muscles in the buttocks and thighs. Begin in a standing position, sideways on your yoga mat, with your feet wide apart and your heels aligned. This is the starting position for the yoga pose Warrior II. Make sure that the toes on your right foot are facing up toward the top of the mat by rotating that foot outward.

Raise your arms until they are level with your shoulders and parallel to the ground. Make sure they are positioned over your legs with your palms facing upward. As you exhale, bend your front knee and make sure it stays aligned over the top of your foot while you do so. Maintain a straight position across the middle of your body and turn your head such that you are looking over your right hand. Maintain this position for one full minute. The process is then repeated on the opposite side.

This position strengthens the cardiovascular system and activates the abdominal muscles. Additionally, the groin, chest, and shoulders are all opened up as a result.

13. Tree Pose Or Vrksasana

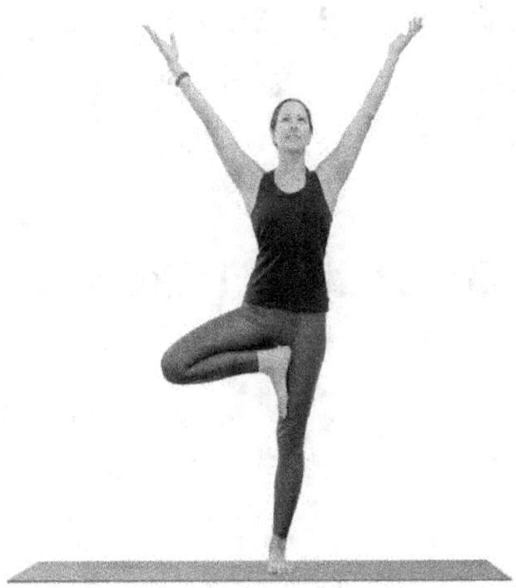

Maintain your balance by standing on one foot and planting it firmly on the ground. Put the other foot up against your thigh or calf (not your knee), and make sure that your toes are pointing down toward the ground. Your hips should be in a square position, and your pelvis should maintain its centered position.

You can either bring your hands to the middle of your chest or stretch your arms upward.
A yogi can improve their sense of balance and strengthen their thighs, ankles, and spine by practicing this pose.

14. Triangle Or Utthita Trikonasana

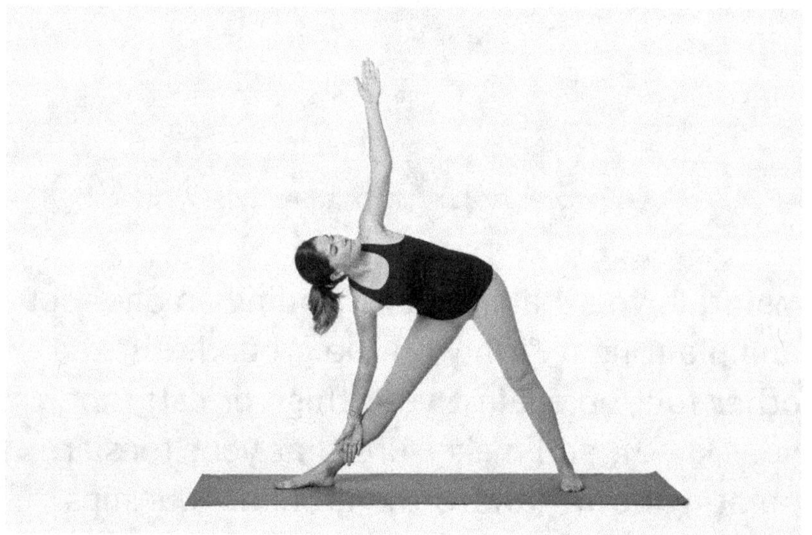

To begin, stand with your feet approximately four feet apart from one another.

Put your arms out to the side so that they are perpendicular to the ground. Then, bring one hand down toward your foot and grip either your ankle or your shin (if you are flexible enough, you can also rest your hand on the floor at this point). The other one of your hands should be raised up toward the heavens. Keep your focus on the sky above your fingertips.

The legs are toned, and there is increased stability throughout the lower body as a result of this stance. Additionally, it provides a profound stretch for the hamstrings, hips, and back.

15. High Plank Or Kumbhakasana

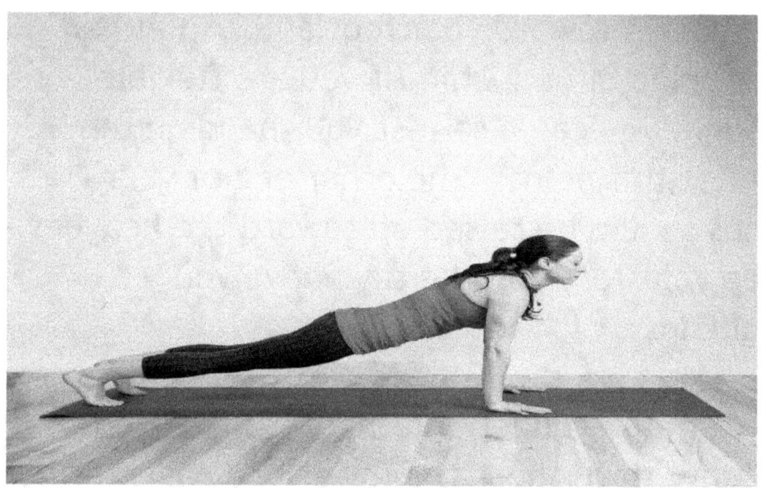

Begin by getting down on your hands and knees. Put your wrists in a position where they are directly under your shoulders. Spread your fingers apart and apply downward pressure with both hands. Take a step backward and tuck your toes before bringing your legs off the mat in a standing position. Consolidate your muscles and try to widen your shoulders.

Achieve a position in which your chest is directly over your hands.

This pose is beneficial for building arm and core strength; nevertheless, it is important to remember not to allow your hips to fall too low.

16. Standing Fold Or Uttanasana

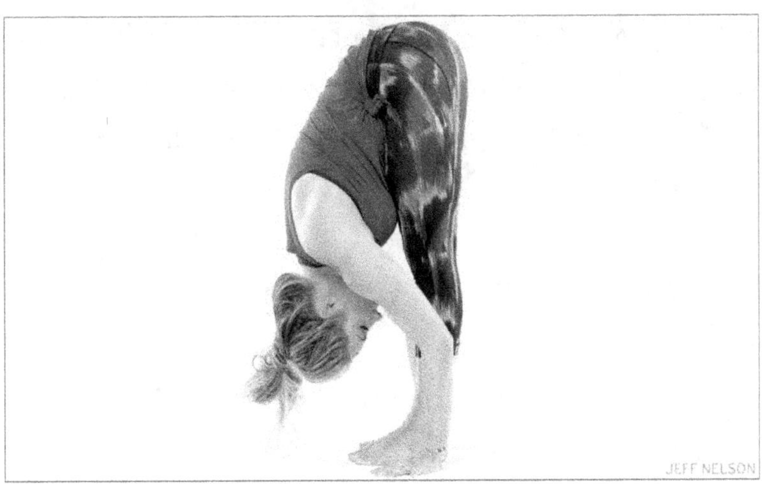

Maintain a confident stance with your hands resting on your hips. Forward bending starts from the hips. As you move lower, make sure to lengthen your torso. If you are able to do so, place your palms or the tips of your fingers on the ground in front of you (or as far as you can reach). You can either keep your legs completely straight or gently bend them.

In between holding other positions in your practice, you should try to relax into this stress-relieving posture to help calm the mind. In addition to that, it helps strengthen the thighs and knees.

Don't Be Scared

When you first begin practicing yoga, it is important to pay attention to how your body feels and to go at your own pace.

Try not to be too hard on yourself if you find that you can't quite get your foot in between your hands when performing the Revolving Crescent Lunge or if you lose your balance when performing a Side Plank. You are going to arrive there at some point. If you maintain your practice, you will notice that your body will start to want yoga as time goes on. Your mind will be more at ease, and the stiffness that you've been feeling in your joints will become a distant memory. You'll also have better sleep.